I0428967

Achieve Better vision In 30 Days!

By Amir K. Campbell

Table Of Contents

Disclaimer

I'm not a medical doctor and these techniques are not intended to be cures. I offer them to you the reader as an alternative approach to corrective vision. Please make sure you go to a qualified ophthalmologist before you perform any of the exercises in this manual to determine your individual level of vision impairment. Once the eye doctor has given you the diagnosis, then you can focus on the appropriate steps to correct your vision.

Chapter 1: Why Do Our Eyes "go bad"?

Remember when you were younger and you could see everything as clear as crystal? Well, some of us have always had good vision and some of us, not so much. I've been fortunate to always have good vision. Some of my fondest memories as a child are of me lying on back under the Mid-July sky, looking up at the blue sky and attempting to pierce that veil to see outer space. I was always a weird kid, and it made life pretty fun.

I can remember the day when I started my quest to find natural methods for both myself and my family to stay healthy and remain healthy: My mother had just had cataract surgery. She's Caribbean and she looks very young for her 62 year old self. I remember the huge black glasses that she had to wear to protect her hyper-dilated eyes from the glare of the winter sun bouncing off of the snow. I was curious as to why there weren't any medications her doctor could give her to prevent her from having the surgery and fixing her eyes. At this time in my life, I was deeply interested in meditation and the subconscious mind. Everything I'd read up to that point said that most imbalances in the body are caused by improper diet and improper thoughts and beliefs. Of course, environmental factors, like being out in blazing sunlight without the proper eye wear, can play a part in why our eyes go "bad", and we can address those as well.

If you look at my last sentence closely, you'll notice an example of a negative thought pattern: How is it possible that my eyes can "go bad"? Because words are so powerful, do you think it's possible that thinking of my eyes as bad can have a negative effect on the cells that make up my eyes? I do, and apparently, science does as well. There have been scientific studies down that show that the emotional states that a person experiences are instantly reverberated in the cells of their body – even when the person and their cells are separated by miles of distance! Edgar Cayce, the great American psychic, stated that a person cannot hate their neighbor and not experience any negative side effects in their stomachs. The power of the mind-body connection has been known for centuries, but in our day and age, we tend to cover over that power with the power of medicine. Don't get me wrong, you better believe that if I have some sort of ache or pain that I can't explain away or visualize away I will be taking aspirin, especially after a really intense week of personal training and possibly a set of Tabata high intensity interval protocols!

In addition to old age, our eyesight tends to dim because of improper diet. You're going to learn some simple dietary tricks that you can begin using today to build stronger eyes.

Like any muscle, our eyes tend to get lose and flabby if we

don't give them proper exercise AND proper rest. You're going to learn how to do exactly that in this book.

As mentioned before, negative thoughts trigger negative emotions that release negative energy and adversely affect the subject of our negative judgment. If you want to take the mind-body stuff out of the equation, then open your mind for a moment and think about it like this: Your thoughts are electrical signals and your cells work by electricity: isn't it logical for you to assume that an electric spark in one part of the system can fry another part?

You're going to learn simple and powerful ways to install positive beliefs into your neurology so that you start to see better immediately.

One reason that most people don't consider as a cause of diminished eyesight is high blood pressure. High blood pressure is cause by many things, particularly stress, and while this is not the focus of this book, you're going to learn simple ways to relax and releases stress from your body.

Be joyous and excited for the prospect of new vision!!!

Chapter 2: How Bad Do You Want It?

Depending on the severity of your vision impairment, you will either see quick or slow improvements in your vision. But have hope, because with consistent practice, you will improve your vision. A reasonable time frame within which to see amazing results is about 30 days. You may be able to toss your glasses away for good or your may simply be able to reduce the use of said spectacles. Either way, your vision will get better.

Think about it like this:

When you go on a road trip, you have a destination in mind, don't you? If you have no destination then how can you possibly know where you're going? In that case, you won't know where you are until you get there and then it may totally suck.

On a deeper level, keeping this subtle intention of better vision in the back of your mind as you the exercises will unlock powerful healing forces inside just waiting to get moving.

Most importantly, please remember that none of the exercises in this manual will work for you if you don't use them. Give each exercise a go, and see which ones work better for you. If you're doing an exercise you notice instant improvements in your vision, keep using it. However, I guarantee that you'll be using every exercise whenever you can, because many of them have more than one benefit. Have fun☺

Tap into the power of gratitude

Gratitude is a very powerful healing force that we all have access to. One of the best ways to start healing your vision is to be thankful for the vision that you have right now! It could be worse, you could be completely blind. It could be worse; you could only have vision in one eye. It could be worse; you could have no color vision whatsoever. You get the picture.

In order to tap into the deep reserves of gratitude energy laying in wait for you in your Heart Chakra, perform the following:

1. Take a few deep breaths, inhaling through your nose and exhale through your mouth. As you breathe, relax

your abdomen and focus on your breathing.

2. Place your hands on your heart chakra, on the spot right over your heart.

3. As you rest your hands on your heart chakra, the 4th of the seven major chakras located in the human body, mentally say thank you to your eyes.

4. You can even verbally express your gratitude for your eyes. Be thankful that you can see right now.

Chapter 3: Why do YOU want to See Better?

Before we go any further, I want you stop for a moment, and list five reasons why you want to see better and clearer. Remember, your own reasons are YOUR own reasons, no matter how they may sound to others. Your reasons will give you the motivation to do the drills in this book. Every time you feel like you don't want to do the drills, think about your reasons for wanting to see clearer. Think about how much money you'll be saving on contact lenses. Think about how much pain you'll avoid once you're able to reduce how much time you spend wearing your glasses. You're going to write down your reasons (find as many as possible) and keep them someplace where you can see them every day. You can make copies of your reasons and place them in those places (I.e. Office desk, Work station, etc)

I want you to think about how much better your life will be

when your vision has improved. What types of things will you be doing when your vision is better? Will you feel more confident moving about in your daily life, navigating this modern day jungle?

Chapter 4: Trying on your new pair of eyes

I want you to close your eyes... and imagine that your vision is perfect and you can see clearly. Now... what's it like now that your vision is better?

What types of things can you see clearly?

I want you to imagine that your standing or sitting outside on a warm, sunny day... you're in a place that you really enjoy spending time and you're completely relaxed...Now... as you look around, what types of things do you see going around? As you see these things going on around you now, you find that you can easily zoom in and focus on colors. Zoom in on a color that attracts your attention and really notice it. How bright is it? Can you determine what color it is? As you notice how that color is, you start to realize that your vision is becoming better and better...

The purpose of the above exercise is sort of "try on" the eyesight you want to experience. It will allow you to remember what you are working towards when you use the techniques presented here. This is called Mental Rehearsal. It's something that people do every day, whether consciously or unconsciously. Mental rehearsal can be used to improve athletic performance and you've seen (pun intended) it can be used to both communicate with your subconscious mind and receive information from it.

Another purpose of doing the process above is to move your mind from the problem back to your Motivation. Sure, you probably can't see all that good yet, but do you WANT to see better? There's an important distinction there.

I'll take this moment to remind you again to physically write out your goals for better vision to help you keep your laser focused concentration on moving towards better vision. Another important reason for you to write out ANY goals is because the simple act of writing them out increases your compliance and commitment by 44%; in other words, written goals are more likely to be achieved than goals that are just allowed to float around in your mind and compete with the psychic maelstrom therein. Writing goals down is the equivalent of creating a powerful pull, keeping you totally focused on your goal.

The first is noticing the problem or challenge. The next step is to find ways to change the situation and get what we want.

Getting this manual is only the first step. You'll need to put in daily effort if you want to see better and clearly. Have you ever tried to use a blender by just staring at it? If you ever figure out how to do that, teach me how. Chances are however, that the blender ain't going anywhere until you actually get up, walk over to it, plug it in, make sure it's working, put your ingredients in the blender, put the lid on, and stand back and watch the magic.

It's the exact same thing with this manual you're reading here: sure, you have a bunch of effective techniques for improving your vision, but are you going to use them? Or are you going to just keep this book and not use the techniques in here? The choice is yours, but if you're smart then you already know that you have to APPLY these techniques for them to help you. You have to put pressure on the gas pedal before you can MOVE FORWARD, right?

Since you're reading this now, I'm going to go out on a limb and just guess that you'd like to improve your ability to see objects at both a distance and up close, right?

Speaking of reading, reading for long periods of time without rest is a common cause of eyestrain. Whenever you have to read a book or something for whatever reason, look up from time to time and focus on some object in the distance. Take the time to really focus in on that distant object and rest your eyes from that narrow focus required for reading. Our eyes are designed to see RELAXED and at great distances. Reading is a strain on them.

Vision is very important for many reasons, most of all survival. We use vision all day, every day to assess threats and even choose the people we like to...get to know better...with :) Vision is one of the three highly developed senses in Humans, along with touch and hearing. We rely on our eyesight to help us distinguish friend from foe. They help us determine if that stick we were about to step on is actually a stick...or a venomous snake. We rely on our vision to help us determine distance and width. Vision is an important aspect of daily life and it's important that it's is function at peak capacity, wouldn't you agree?

The ability to see clearly is something that most people take for granted, and there are people out there who would love to be able to see clearly without the use of glasses or contacts.

On a much deeper level, vision is necessary for DIRECTION. Without vision, you'll be stuck doing things that you don't like doing, or worse... You need vision so that you can move forward towards the things that you WANT, and move away from the things that you don't want.

If I told you that there are tested and proven methods to help you see better in a month or less, would you want to learn them?

Of course you would!!! In fact, I know you're just chomping at the bit to learn the techniques so you can heal your eyesight right now!!! In this manual, you're going to learn simple processes that can help see better than you have in years.

There are lots of causes that contribute to decreased efficiency, one of which is stress. Stress in daily life can cause tension, and tension contributes to a reduced ability to see properly. Vision is normally a passive event, meaning that you shouldn't have to strain in order to see something.

Have you ever seen people squinting to look at something in the distance or even something right in front of them? Well, that's unnatural. In a person with healthy eyesight, just the intention to see what's going on up ahead or right in front of you is enough to adjust the lens of your eyes to fit your desire, without squinting or furrowing your eyebrows as in deep concentration.
 By consciously relaxing your mind and relaxing the muscles around your eyes, you set the way to help see better.

When you're stressed and tensed up, your body is in what's called "fight or flight" mode, which is the term for a set of physiological processes that occur in the body with one intention in mind: To help you survive. When you're in fight or flight mode, your body releases adrenaline, which prepares you to face the threat or run from it. In some cases, your body will actually freeze to the spot. This natural set of processes is EXACTLY what you to happen when you're faced with danger, like a huge black bear chasing you down. In this case, you want all the adrenaline your body can secrete to give you the speed to haul ass.

However, here's the thing about the fight or flight response: It's triggered by seemingly little things that occur in daily life, like driving home during rush hour traffic, or thinking about the argument you had last night with your girlfriend/boyfriend. I personally believe that these incidences aren't life threatening, as you can easily find a new girlfriend/boyfriend. You can easily find ways to relax so instead of feeling like your crossing the desert on your hands and knees during that evening commute home, you can feel like you being driven home by a chauffeur. Isn't that a nice way to feel?

Having said that, you, being the intelligent person that you are, can see where I'm going with this, can't you? Of course you can!! You were thinking," ...well, if stress and tension contribute to decreased eyesight, then being relaxed can help me to see better..." right?

One simple way to help you relax is to practice deep, diaphragmatic breathing. Deep breathing not only allows your body to draw lots of fresh, life giving oxygen, but it also helps you to relax, and relaxation offers you much good benefits. Being able to relax in social settings and other situations allows you to be present wherever you are and fully appreciate and experience what's going on around. In addition, you might find it interesting to know that your brain uses One Fifth of the oxygen your body consumes, and that your eyes are actually projections on your brain. WOW....

A benefit that many people don't realize at first is that people will enjoy being around you, because you radiate a relaxed and confident vibe that's contagious. I'm not sure how that can help you out in your daily life.

Deep breathing acts as a reset button for your nervous system, allowing you to drain all that tension you've accumulated. For now, you can think of your nervous system as a rubber band, and you can think of stress as the tension that you apply to the rubber band. As we go through the day, we tend to stretch that rubber band tighter and tighter. When you learn to breathe deeply and properly, you can reset the tension in your rubber band (nervous system), so you can start fresh. Isn't that awesome?

I wonder if you can use that little bit of knowledge BEFORE and AFTER your exercise session to be stronger and play longer... Hmmm....

You're going to learn a very simple rhythmic breathing pattern that will allow you to relax and enjoy yourself wherever you be, not to mention give you much needed shot of energy. It's very simple, and you can do it anywhere you want once you get the breathing pattern down. Well get to that in a moment...

What you're going to learn now is very important, not just for vision enhancement, but for health and vitality. It's a drill called "freeing the diaphragm" and it's designed to increase circulation and pump oxygen throughout your entire body. Having good circulation is crucial to vision, as the eyes and the brain need a steady supply of blood and oxygen to work at their best. In addition, many studies have been done which prove that cancer cannot survive in an environment that is oxygenated. By doing the diaphragm drill, you'll pump life giving oxygen throughout your entire body.

The diaphragm is a strong, thin shelf of muscle partitioning the chest from the abdomen. It fans oxygen throughout the body. The following exercise helps distribute oxygen to every cell, gland, and organ. Here's what you're going to do:

1) Firmly place your left hand under the center of your ribcage and place your right hand on top of it. With your hands flat, pull your elbows close to your body so you are hugging your midsection.

2) Inhale deeply and push your body toward your hands while your hands push back against your body. Hold your breath and push hard. Although there is no set amount of time, the longer you hold your breath and push (without becoming light headed), the better.

3) Release your breath naturally, along with your hands.

4) Relax. Do two more times.

This exercise is a good one to do in the mornings or anytime you just want to relax. You can think of this drill as a sort of warm up, as it releases your diaphragm if it's stuck, so now whenever you take a deep breath, life giving oxygen is sent coursing through every part of your body. Isn't that amazing...

A powerful deep breathing exercise for more energy and better eyesight!

Now, let's move onto the breathing exercise, the main course, if you will :)

First, if you're driving a very long distance, you'll want to pull over to the side of the road for a moment. Obviously, this is NOT something that you want to do while driving on the road. It is, however, perfectly okay to pull over and do the breathing, so that way you can start your journey fresh with energy and a clear mind. As a general rule, it's perfectly safe to do this anywhere you can sit down for a moment and relax, preferably by yourself. When you practice and get really good at this, you can do it in front of others and still relax deeply.

First, you're going to close your eyes for a moment. That's it, just allow your eyes to shut and allow them to relax. Feel the muscles around your eyes relax. You can just imagine them relaxing completely. It's easy to do this, because our body responds most readily to our thoughts. Imagine a feeling of warmth and relaxation flowing around your eye muscles. Tell that part of your body to relax and let go. You're going to focus your attention on your body and you're going to notice any areas of tension. When you feel a place that's tense, you're going to allow it to relax. Don't try to relax it, because the more you try to relax, the harder it becomes. Instead, you're simply going to tell your body that it can relax completely. It's totally safe to relax where you are. Start from the top of your head and work your way down to the bottoms of your feet.

As you notice any tension, simply tell that part of your body to relax.

Now.... Here comes the fun stuff, the stuff you've been waiting for. You going to take a deep breath, and let it out through the mouth. This breath is sort of like priming a pump, a relaxation pump. That one simple deep breath is like flipping the relaxation switch, so now when you take another deep breath, you can relax even deeper.

Now, here comes the actual breathing pattern. You're going to inhale for 4 seconds, hold that inhalation for about 4 seconds, and then, you going to release that exhalation though your mouth, slowly and gently. It helps if you make an "ahhh" sound as you exhale to help you release it slowly.

As you sit there with your eyes closed, breathing in this way, you can even bring to mind a mental picture that makes you relax and feel good. It doesn't matter what it is, so long as it causes you to feel good when you think about it. In fact, it doesn't even have to be a mental picture, it can be a sound, or a smell, or even a simple affirmation. The important thing is that it helps you to feel good. This simple technique will allow you to automatically activate your relaxation response.

You can sit there and relax as long as you like, and when you feel ready to do so, you can open your eyes, smile, and go on with your day.

The very awesome thing about his process is that the more you practice it, the quickly you'll be able to relax. It becomes a conditioned response, so your body is becoming conditioned to relax deeply anytime you take a few deep breaths. It usually takes about 21 to 30 days for a desired response to become conditioned into your neurology, so daily practice is necessary if you want to make relaxation a part of your daily life.

How much easier will it be to deal with your employees and

even you're FAMILY when you're deeply relaxed and centered?

This is an excellent breathing technique to do right before you step out of the car and head toward the doors of your home. As I mentioned before, emotional states are contagious, so what do think will happen when you walk through the door, totally relaxed and glowing? How is that different from walking through the door, pissed off at the guy that just cut you off in traffic or pissed off at that coworker that did that thing again that you really hate?

Oh, and in case you're still curious as to how deep breathing can benefit your eyes, keep in mind that your brain requires sufficient oxygen to do its job. Do you remember what I said about our eyes are like the "fingers" of our brains? Our eyes are essentially the visible portion of our brains. When you feed the brain with oxygen, you in turn feed the eyes with the oxygen they need to do the job they were meant to do.

As a matter of fact, this is an excellent way to start the day. If you work long hours doing lots of complex mental work like editing or even physical activity, it's a good way to fill your body up with oxygen and consequently, energy to meet the demands of your particular occupation.

If you need any clarification whatsoever on the above process, then please feel free to email me so I can help you understand the process better.

Chapter 6: The Power Of Healing In Your Hands

Let's move on another technique which is excellent for correcting vision problems. It's called "palming", and essentially, what it does is provide a much needed rest for your eyes. It was discovered by a man named William H. bates, a very skilled ophthalmologist. He discovered many things about the mechanics of vision and created many processes for correcting vision. One such technique is the aforementioned Palming. He became aware of something very important concerning the eyes:

Even though they might be closed, the eyes can still be stimulated by external light sources. The eyes can only rest in complete darkness. He devised a simple method which will allow a person to completely rest their eyes, so the eyes can adjust themselves naturally. He also discovered something very interesting and crucial to the mechanics of the palming technique:

He discovered that people had a tendency to see colored lights whenever they palmed or even closed their eyes. He made an even more amazing correlation: The brighter the visual disturbances, the more damaged the person's vision was. This feedback allows a person to know exactly how much progress they are making as you use this technique.

If you want to fix your vision, you can start to use the palming technique right now and see results immediately, especially when you add a few more processes which I'll be sharing with you in a moment.

Here's the exact palming procedure, in the words of William Bates himself:

"All the methods used in the eradication of errors of refraction are simply different ways of obtaining relaxation, and most people, though by no means all, find it easiest to relax with their eyes shut. This usually lessen the strain to see, and in such cases is followed by a temporary or more lasting improvement in vision.

Most people are benefitted merely by closing the eyes; and by alternately resting them for a few minutes or longer in this way and then opening them and looking at a test card for a second or less, flashes of improved vision are as a rule very quickly obtained. Some temporarily obtain almost normal vision by this means, and in rare cases a complete restoration has been effected, sometimes in less than an hour.

But some light comes through the closed eye lids, and a still greater degree of relaxation can be obtained, in all but a few exceptional cases, by excluding it. This is done by covering the eyes with the palms of the hands without putting pressure on the eyes whatsoever (the fingers resting on the head)..."

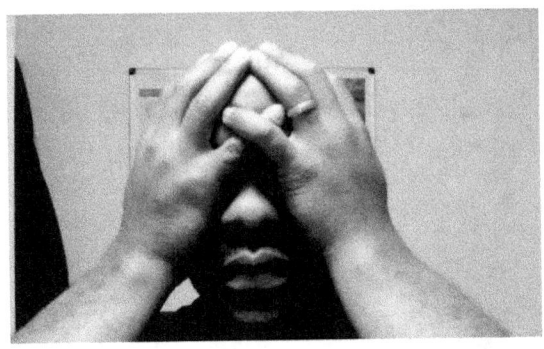

Palming the eyes for complete relaxation and rejuvenation.

The method is very effective, especially when you combine it with the rhythmic breathing exercise you're learning. The combination of palming with rhythmic breathing will allow you to relax completely as your eyes are relaxing completely. Bates discovered that everyone can see nearly perfectly when they are they completely relaxed. He also discovered that if a person were to remember something black as they were palming, they could relax their eyes even further and achieve amazing results. This connection between memory, the mind and the body is so awesome and awe inspiring, isn't it?

Bates recommends that you remember some familiar black object, preferably something that you see every day and can clearly visualize, like a black cat, or a black leather coat, etc. You can think of all the black objects that you can visualize as you palm.

One interesting side note: Bates cites an example where a man palmed for 24 hours straight, drinking nothing but water. Before palming, this man required glasses for both seeing objects at a distance and for reading up close. However, after 24 hours of palming, his vision was restored to normal and remained that way permanently. Now, I'm not advising that you palm for this length of time, as it's not necessary, however, if you can find 2 minutes a day to palm and do your breathing, you will see results quickly, especially when start to incorporate the other techniques I'll be providing in this manual. The best times to palm are:

1) In the morning, as you're laying there in bed.
2) In the evening, as your laying down in bed, getting ready to fall asleep.

The beauty of this technique is that you can use it anytime, anywhere. You can use it at work in your office or cubicle, and you can even palm in the bathroom, if you can bear the smell... I palm every morning before starting my work, as I find it helps me clear my head and get ready to face the rest of the day. As an added benefit of palming, you actually have your fingers on very important points called neurovasculars. These neurovasculars bring blood to specific areas and organs of the body. In this position, you are bringing blood to your liver.

In order to supercharge your palming and increase your energy and vitality as well, perform the relaxation breathing exercise given previously.

1. Take up a comfortable position and begin palming.
2. As you're in the position, practice the following breathing exercise: Inhale for 4 seconds, hold for 4 seconds, exhale for 4 seconds, and hold your lungs empty for 4 seconds.
3. Repeat this breathing pattern for 5 minutes.

When you make this simple change to the already powerful technique of palming, you will increase the amount of oxygen that you get to your brain and improve your vision and energy levels at the same time. This technique works so awesomely because the eyes are essentially projections of the brain.

Regarding the breathing exercise: You may notice that you have difficulty keeping up the prescribed pattern for a long period of time and that's ok! This is a signal to you that your lung capacity could sue a little boost. Start with a smaller pattern until you gradually gain the strength to maintain the 4 second rhythm. Some people start with 2 seconds, some people can start with 1. The point is to start where YOU are at and grow from there. You'll eventually get to the point where you can perform a 7-7-7-7 or even a 10-10-10-10 pattern with ease! This is a good sign that your health and vitality are improving and your eyesight is surely getting better by the day.

There's another benefit associated with closing your eyes: Researchers discovered that when a person shuts their eyes, their brainwaves begin to slow down and vibrate at what is called Alpha brainwave, a rate of vibration which is associated with relaxation and daydreaming. This brainwave state is also associated with light states of hypnosis. You can give yourself affirmations and self suggestion in this state. You can program yourself to look for the positive in people or the positive aspects in a situation. You can give yourself any suggestion you like.

Remember, it usually takes between 21 and 30 days to program yourself with new habits. The key ingredient in success is repetition. The more you give yourself the suggestions, the quicker you'll see results. You'll see results immediately; however, if you want that specific habit to stick around, repetition is the key. It's exactly like riding a bike: At first, you weren't so good at it, however, the more you got on that bike and rode it, the better you got at it until it became second nature and now you can ride a bike with even thinking twice. In fact, you might even be able to pull off all those neat tricks. It's the exact same thing with wiring in new habits. Practice makes permanent...

Some sample suggestions are: "My vision is getting sharper and clearer each and every day.... I see farther every day.... I'm starting to see colors clearly..." and so on. Of course, you're going to tailor the suggestions to fit your individual situation, depending on whether or not you're nearsighted or far sighted.

The subconscious mind is moved most deeply by images and sensations. Can you see yourself looking at the objects around with perfectly relaxed vision, picking up the slightest movement and your eyes feel fine and perfectly relaxed...

Now, moving swiftly on....

One very important thing to do that makes a HUGE difference is to appreciate what you are able to see RIGHT NOW. Sure, there are some things that you are seeing with difficulty and your vision isn't where you want it to be YET, and you need to realize that YOU CAN SEE RIGHT NOW and BE THANKFUL. Many people are in the habit of cursing themselves and their temporary conditions, and they fail to realize that they are actually making things WORSE!!!

Much scientific research has been done on the influence of our thoughts and feelings over our bodies, organs and cells and everything in between. Educational kinesiology can be used to demonstrate the effects of positive and negative thoughts on your strength and the health of your body. In hypnosis terms, praising what you can do already is POSITIVE reinforcement, and cursing yourself for what you can't YET do is negative reinforcement. Keeping in mind that your subconscious mind is responsible for all of your bodily functions, doesn't make sense that you want to give it POSITIVE messages and a positive focus on what you want it to do? If you believe in the Law Of Attraction, Like Me, then you know that you get what you focus on.

Also be aware of the FACT that the mind is indivisible, meaning that you can only focus on one thing at a time. These two ideas are very powerful, especially when you stop to think where in your daily life you can use them. I wonder if you can use them right now…

You're going to learn some "alternative" methods for vision enhancement. The methods that you are going to learn here are based on Chinese medicine and make use of meridians, which are sort of like energy highways in your body. Their job is to carry energy throughout your body and ultimately feed your muscles, bones, organs, and every tissue and cell in your body. Meridians are part of daily conversation in most eastern cultures, however, if you were to ask someone from the United States what a meridian is, they might look at you funny. However, much research has been done on the energy highways that flow through your body. One notable study that verified what traditional Chinese medicine practitioners have been telling us for years:

A very detailed study, involving 330 people, was carried out to determine if the meridians actually existed. The researchers injected a radioactive isotope into an acupuncture point. Having done that, the researchers used a gamma camera to trace the travel path of said isotope. The researchers discovered that the isotope traveled the paths that were associated with the meridians that had been mapped some 4,000 years before by Chinese Doctors.

If you're interested in reading the complete study yourself, you can go here and read it:

http://www.emofree.com/Research/Research-other/meridianexistence.htm

My intention here, however is to provide techniques that work, techniques that when used regularly (remember repetition?) will improve your vision far beyond what it is right now. The proof is in the seeing, is it not? Having said that, let's move on, shall we?

The first set of meridian points that you're going to learn to activate and stimulate is the kidney meridians, specifically the 27th point on the kidney meridian. These points are very important, because when you stimulate these points, you stimulate every other meridian in the body. When you tap and/or rub these points, you cause every other meridian in the body to flow forward in its proper direction. In a nutshell, when the meridians are flowing backward, you experience tiredness, fatigue, an inability to focus, and much, much more. They are located here:

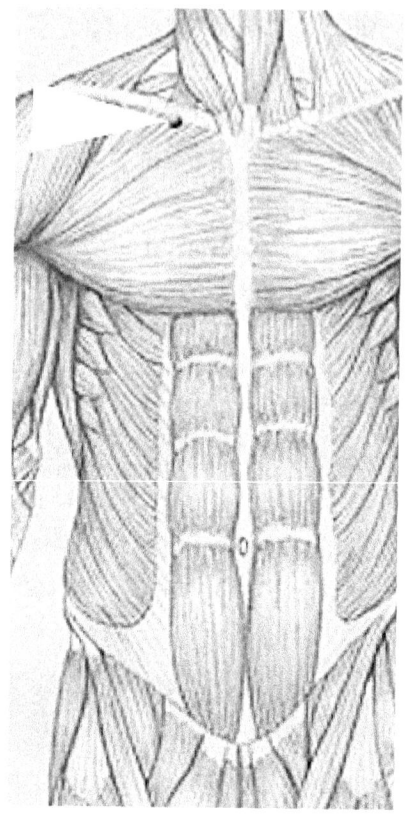

This picture is property of

When the meridians are flowing forward in the direction they were meant to, you experience more energy, more stamina, and your vision is brightened. These points have a direct impact on your vision, as stimulating these points will send energy to straight up to your eyes. If you're interested in learning more about the meridians and how you can optimize their flow for more energy and vitality, then there are literally hundreds of books on the market that can teach you how to do that, however, there is one book that is very easy to understand and you can apply the information in it immediately. It's called "Energy Medicine" and you can find it at any bookstore. You can even find used copies on any online book site that sells used books. It's a very good investment, in my opinion.

To find these points, you're going to put a finger in the notch directly below your throat area, that notch at the top of the sternum (breastbone). There's a u- shaped notch at the top of the breastbone. Once you find that Notch, you're going to move your finger either to the left or right until you are touching the beginning of the collarbone. Now, once you're touching that bone, you're going to move your finger down about an inch. You should now be touching a pad of flesh. When your finger is there, you're going to massage that area. Massage it firmly for about a minute or so. If this area feels sore, then this means YOU REALLY NEED IT. After a few days of massaging that area regularly, the soreness will disappear. Now, here's where it gets fun:

You're going to tap those spots underneath the collarbones. That's right, you read me correct: You're going to tap those points. When you tap those points, you're waking up those points.

Rubbing them is good, but tapping them is even better. Rubbing is like eating cheesecake; Tapping is like eating New York style cheese cake with chocolate and strawberries dripping down the sides, served with a glass of sparkling white wine. Now I'm making myself drool... Tapping will cause every single meridian in your body to flow forward in the proper direction. Your vision will improve, and you'll notice that you're definitely more focused. That's a lot to experience for such a simple exercise, isn't it? Do this exercise anytime during the day, especially when you feel like you're moving uphill, or it just seems like walking forward is a bit of a struggle. When our meridians are flowing properly, you feel as though you're being pushed or supported. Make sense?

Here's a variation on the kidney point tap that will help increase the amount of oxygen to your brain and increase your visual abilities:

1. Place one hand on your navel. This helps you to ground your energy and relax.
2. Take the fingers of your other hand and place them on your kidney points (K-27's).
3. With your hand relaxed on your navel, rub your kidney points for several seconds.
4. Switch hands and repeat.

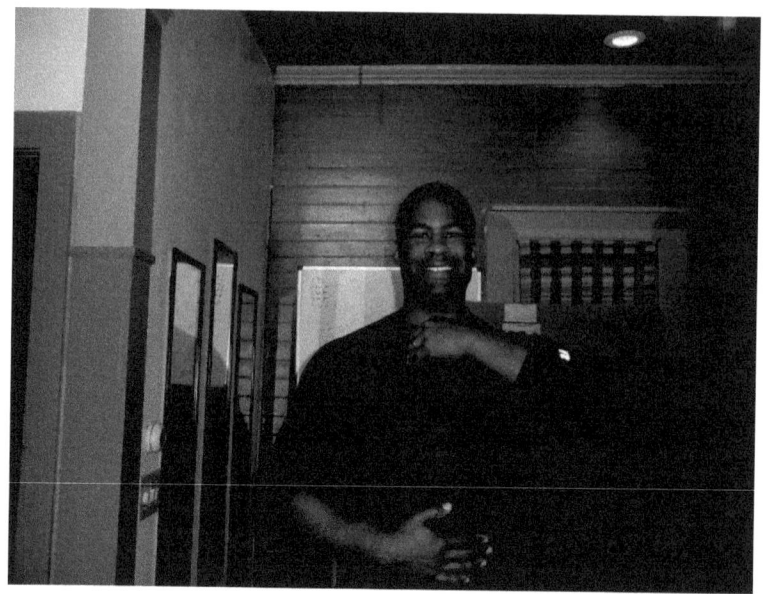

K27's + Navel Variation

Once you've tapped your kidney points get your energies flowing in the proper direction, perform Cross Crawl to improve your binocular vision, further increase your vitality, increase the flow of your lymph, and increase the coordination between the left and right hemispheres of your brain:

1. Seated or standing, raise your left knee as you raise your right arm.

2. Repeat on the other side, raising your right knee and then your right arm.

3. Perform this marching in place as you breathe deeply in through your nose and out through your mouth for about 1 minute.

Another simple technique you can use right now is to tap the meridian endpoints underneath your eyes, which are the end points of the stomach meridian. The stomach meridian also feeds the eyes with energy and when there is a disturbance in that meridian, your vision is impacted. You can stimulate this meridian by tapping on these specific points. You can use the pads of your index and middle fingers to gently tap these points:

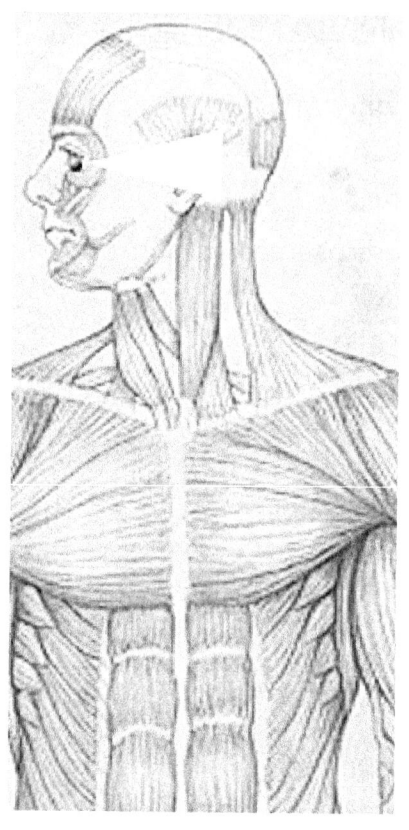

As you tap these points, you're going to say a little affirmation to yourself i.e. "I choose to see clearly... My eyes are relaxing... My vision is getting clearer and clearer everyday..." These are just sample affirmations and you can sit down and think of a few that are specific to your vision concerns. You can either hold these points or tap them, the decision is yours. As you tap those points underneath your eyes, look around you and focus in on the different objects in front of you. It adds

tremendous power to the tapping procedure.

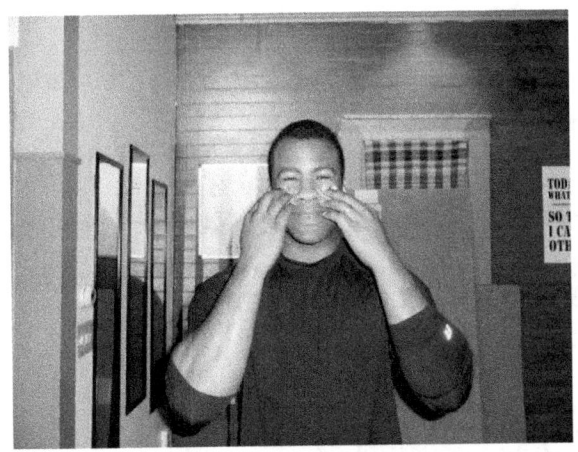

Tapping the stomach points

Another acupressure point that you can use right now to help

enhance your vision is the HOKU point, which is located on

the web of flesh between your thumb and index finger:

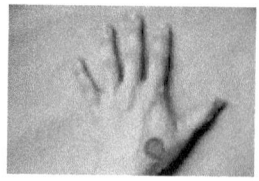

The hoku point, Large intestine 4

In traditional Chinese medicine, the liver is related to vision, and as with the stomach meridian, when there is a disturbance in the energy of the liver meridian, there's a disturbance in the vision/eyesight of the person involved.

This point is related to your liver function (although it is a Large Intestine meridian point) and when you rub this pad of flesh with your thumb, you stimulate your liver and influence your vision. When you first stimulate this point, you might feel some tenderness, and that's perfectly normal. The more you stimulate this point by massaging it whenever you REMEMBER to DO THAT, the more the tenderness will disappear, until that point is no longer tender to the touch. You'll be experiencing two benefits when massage this point: Better Vision and a Healthier liver. This is one that you can do

ANYTIME.

There's another point above the eyebrow in line with the eyeball, which is on the bladder meridian. Tapping these points sends energy to your eyes to help you see better, you can do it as many times a day as you like. First, place your index finger on the point I just described, about one inch above the eyebrow in line with the eyeball. Now, using the index and middle fingers of your free hand, you're going to gently tap the fingertip that's laying on the point above your eyebrow 20-30 times. When you've finished tapping there, you're going to do the same thing with the other eye.

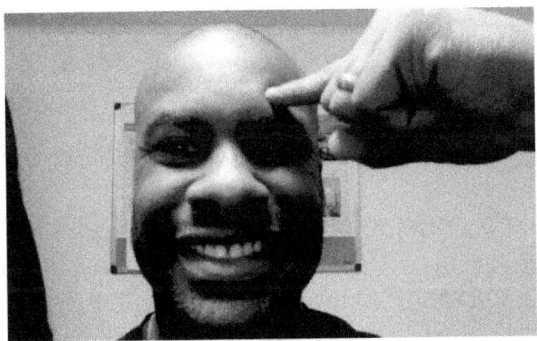

1. Place your index finger on the spot right over your eyeball.

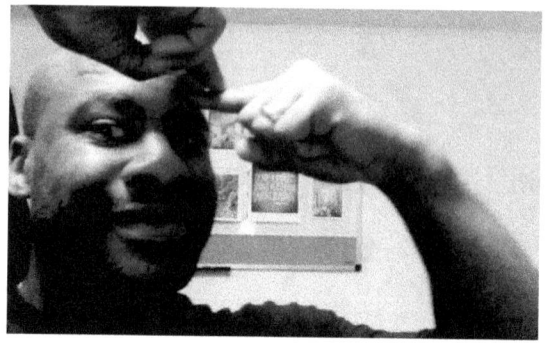

Tapping bladder point for better eyesight.

Used in combination, these simple, easy to follow techniques will enhance your vision in no time. You'll start to notice that you're not using your glasses as much as you used to… and that's perfectly fine. That's the reason why you purchased this manual, isn't it; to see better without the use of glasses or contacts, right?

Good, now let's move on to the next technique you're going to be using. It's a technique discovered by a well known psychic named Edgar Cayce. Edgar Cayce was unique in the sense that he frequently provided remedies for ailments that people were afflicted with. He would frequently provide individuals with strategies for losing weight, regrowing hair, and even…

get ready for it... Fixing your vision. According to Edgar, vision impairment was the result of toxic buildup in the body. He shared a method which will allow a person to restore the circulation of that area of the body, resulting in clearer thinking and of course, BETTER VISION. He recommended that a person do this exercise at least twice a day (Once in the morning when you wake, if you have time and once in the evening when you get home). I'm going to caution you however. If you have ANY preexisting conditions or pains in your cervical neck area, or if you have been diagnosed with osteoporosis, then please IGNORE this exercise. You'll still improve your vision dramatically using all the tips and techniques the manual here.

Here's the exercise:

1) Bend your head forward 3 times, very slowly, and be sure to feel the stretch in the back of your neck muscles.

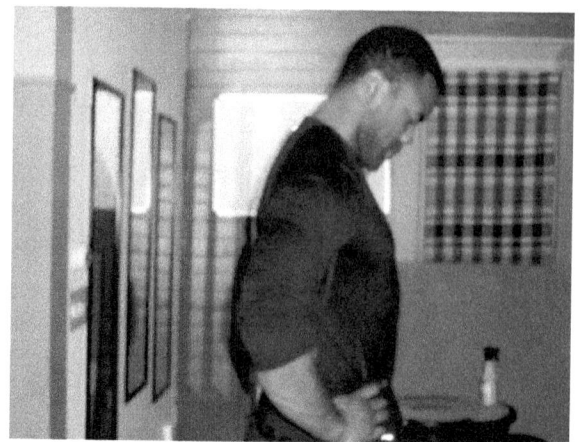

2) Bend your head backward 3 times very slowly, being careful not to force yourself.

3) Bend your head to the right 3 times, slowly, making sure to feel the stretch in your neck muscles.

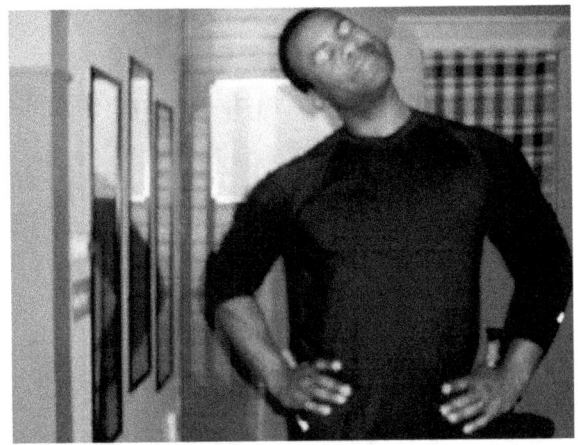

4) Bend your head to the left 3 times, slowly, being sure to feel the stretch in your neck.

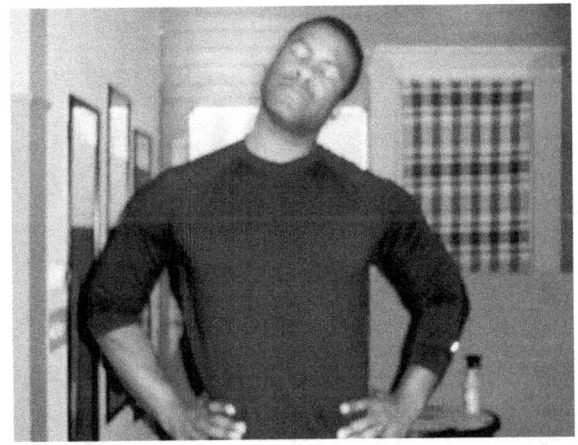

5) Now, rotate your head counterclockwise three times, very slowly.

6) Rotate your head clockwise three times, very slowly.

This is a perfect exercise to do anytime to release tension in your neck area, so feel free to do it more than prescribed.

Clearing your third eye chakra to clear your vision

If you're reading this book and I haven't lost you with all my talk about energies, then keep reading, because it's about to get real. In eastern philosophy, there is the belief that the human body has 7 major chakras, or vortexes, that run up the center of the body. These vortexes are centers wherein which energy is to taken from the universe around us and converted into a format of energy that our physical body uses to function. Each of the seven chakras transforms energy into a different format, depending on its location. These chakras can spin either clockwise or counterclockwise, with the former causing them to absorb energy and the latter causing them to project energy outward.

By spinning a chakra counterclockwise, you can clear the chakra of any gunk that may have accumulated on the surface of it. In the case of clearing your third eye chakra, you'll experience an increase in your mental function, your hearing, your intuition and most importantly, your vision!

In order to clear your third eye chakra, you're going to use the powerful energies coming from your hands to do so. Begin by placing your hand (doesn't matter which one) right in front of the space right between your eyes, called the third eye chakra:

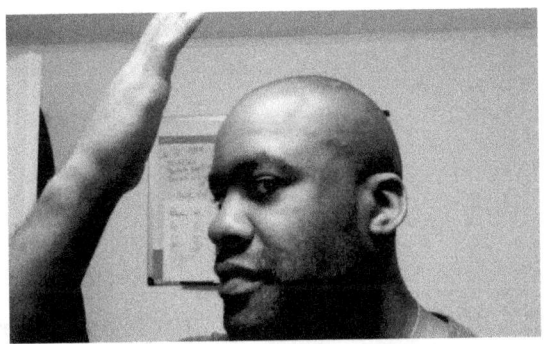

Once you hand is there, begin to circle it in a counterclockwise fashion. Let your body determine which speed feels comfortable to you. Continue circling in this manner for 3 minutes. Once done, shake your hand off and circle it in the clockwise direction for 3 minutes.

The counterclockwise motions helps your body to bring all those gunky energies up to the surface so they can be expelled where as the clockwise motion tells the chakra to spin normally so that it can take in fresh energies.

If you're curious about how you can maximize your performance in daily life by tapping into the power of your chakras, check out the books "The Chakras" by C.W. Leadbeater and "Energy Medicine" By Donna Eden.

Tracing Central Meridian to improve your eyesight.

You've probably noticed by now, but I think Chinese medicine and meridians are awesome, which is why I'm, going to share with you another meridian based way to increase your vision and overall energy levels. This technique is called the Central Meridian Trace. I'll explain central meridian and its importance to the health of your body, mind and spirit: The central meridian is a collection of acu-points that run up the center of the body, starting from the pubic bone and ending right at the dent beneath your lower lip. Central Meridian, or Conception Vessel as it's known in Traditional Chinese medicine, is made up of 24 points.

Although having this meridian flow in the proper direction is crucial for the overall health and integrity of your energy system, our concern here is its relation to vision. The conception vessel, when flowing properly, shoots energy up the center of the body, right to the brain and the eyes.

In order to experience the eye brightening and brain brightening effects of Central meridian, perform the following:

1. Begin with the Kidney Point thump. This will ensure that all of your meridians are flowing properly and will also

give you an energetic boost.

2. Place your hands right on your pubic bone and take a
   deep breath in through your nose and out through your
   mouth.

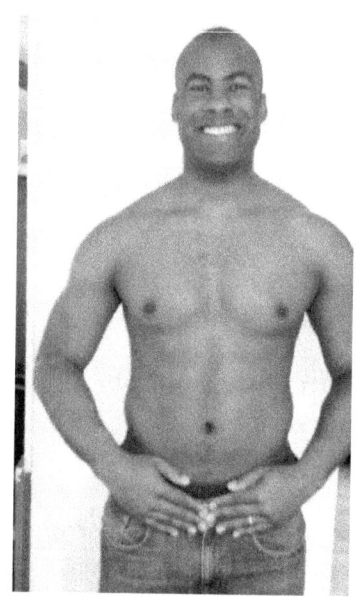

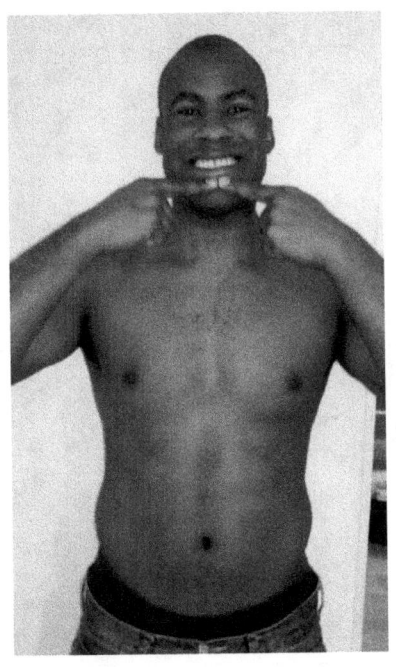

With your hands and fingertips, trace a line moving your hands up from your pubic bone along the centerline of your body, ending at the point right below your bottom lip.

Repeat this tracing sequence 4 more times by moving your hands back to your pubic bone and beginning again.

3. As you trace central meridian, verbally or mentally say to yourself "My eyes are filling with healing energy" or " My eyesight is getting better every day". Find an affirmation that vibes with you and use it every time you zip up.

The 3 step process of tapping your kidney points, marching in place, and tracing your central meridian is a good habit to help you stay energized throughout your day.

Taking the bite out of your triple warmer for better vision

You're probably wondering "what the hell is a triple warmer and why is it biting me without my permission!?!?!?" I'll tell you what it is and I'll tell you why it's probably been biting you your entire life. Triple warmer meridian is one the 12 meridians that flows throughout the body. This particular meridian governs our adrenal and thyroid glands. When we experience stressful circumstances, this meridian begins to suck energy from all of the other meridians except for the heart meridian, because it wants you to live. As a result, it can influence our stress levels. When we get stressed out, our vision tends to narrow. By consciously sedating this meridian, you can reduce your stress responses and experience expanded, relaxed vision. Here's how you can take control and experience awesome vision:

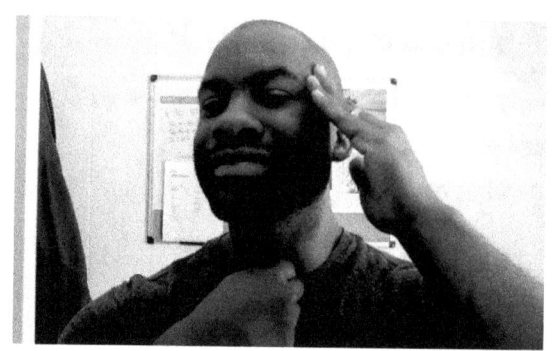

1. Bunch your index, middle (fingers) and thumb of your right hand together to form what we call a 3 finger notch.

2. Take the fingers of your left hand and place them right on your temples.

3. Take 5 deep breaths while in this position, inhaling for 3 seconds, holding for 5, and releasing for 3 seconds.

4. Repeat the holding and the breathing pattern with the hands switched.

With this simple process, you will reduce your fight or flight response and experience more energy and greatly expanded vision, particularly your farsight. As an added spiritual benefit, you may notice that your "see things before they happen" will dramatically increase.

Putting the acupressure techniques together

So you now have a whole slew of acupressure techniques that you can put together to experience greater eyesight. To get the maximal benefit from this program, start by sedating the liver meridian first. This will ensure that you stimulate a fresh flow of energy through that meridian and it will set the pace for the rest of the acupressure work you'll be doing. I would sedate the liver meridian until you start to see vision improvement. This is energy work, so there's nothing you can do to harm yourself.

The triple warmer sedation technique can be done as often as you feel that you need it, especially if you're high stress/highly strung person.

Chapter 8: The role of nutrition on Better eyesight

We all love to eat, right? You damn sure better!!! As your eyes get stronger and your vision gets clearer, they are going to demand more nutrients. Good health and good vision go hand in hand, and to obtain good health, it makes sense that you want to eat good, wholesome food, right? Right. Linus Pauling, a very smart man, one of few people to win MULTIPLE Nobel Peace Prizes by HIMSELF, spent his life researching the effects of various substances on the body, especially vitamin C. He was a brilliant scientist, beginning his career in Quantum Physics. He made some amazing discoveries in this area, particularly that the eye has a significant amount of Vitamin C in it, which means that we need vitamin C to maintain health, and good vision. He suggested a regimen which he was convinced would help people achieve optimum health. He himself lived to the age of 93, and gave lectures up until that time, in sound mind and body. He believed that a lifelong regimen of health should be easy to adhere to; otherwise a person might not want to follow it. Here's his regimen as outlined in his book "How to Live Longer and Feel Better":

1) Take Vitamin C every day.
2) Take Vitamin E every day.
3) Take a B complex everyday
4) Take a Multivitamin every day.
5) Keep your intake of ordinary sugar (sucrose, raw sugar, brown sugar, honey) low. Do not add sugar to tea or coffee. Do not eat high sugar foods. Avoid sweet

deserts. Do not drink soft drinks (sorry).

6) Except for avoiding sugar, eat what you like – but not too much of one food. Eggs and meat are good foods. Also, you should eat some vegetables and fruits. Do not eat so much as to become obese.

7) Drink plenty of water every day. Your kidneys need lots of water to function properly.

8) Keep active; take some exercise daily. Do not at anytime exert yourself physically to an extent far beyond what you are accustomed to (unless you are under the supervision of a qualified personal fitness trainer). Note: 15-30 minutes of activity a day is a good starting point. Find activities that you enjoy and schedule them into your daily routine. If possible, you can take the steps instead the elevator. Think of ways to get more physical activity into your day. The increased blood circulation and oxygen intake will benefit your brain and your eyesight.

9) Drink alcoholic beverages only in moderation. Learn to listen to your body and know when you've had enough.

10) DO NOT SMOKE CIGARETTES. It's been scientifically proven that the chemicals form cigarette smoke can damage the blood vessels in your eyes. Not a good thing if you want perfect sight, right?

11) *Avoid Stress. Work at job you like. Be happy with your family*

Note: There were originally 12 steps in Pauling's original regimen, but I omitted one step, the one in which Pauling recommends that a person take a vitamin A supplement every day. I don't agree with this because Vitamin A is a fat soluble vitamin and can reach toxic levels in liver. If you want to get adequate amounts of Vitamin A, which is essential for normal vision, then eat more colorful fruits and vegetable: Carrots, Peppers, Broccoli, Pumpkin, Spinach, etc. Vitamin C and Vitamin B are water soluble vitamins, and they get excreted every time you go tinkle. B2 (riboflavin) is what makes your tinkle that bright neon color, like a neon sign on the Vegas strip.

Another very powerful aid in your quest for eagle vision is omega fatty acids. Not only do they increase blood circulation (and thus, nutrient delivery to your eyes), protein synthesis, and glucose tolerance, but they also help protect you from macular degeneration. While there is debate as to whether supplementation or eating nutrient dense foods is better for getting nutrients, my stance is this: whatever is convenient for you is the logical choice. Because of the principle of bio-individuality, what works for me nutrition-wise may not be the best approach for you.

(A) No. 11 is unrealistic in my opinion. We are human beings and we experience stress every day, in some way or another. More appropriately, find ways to deal with stressful situations, like exercise, deep breathing (from the diaphragm), meditation, dealing with the people involved in the stressful situation, etc. There are lots of very good books with techniques that will help you manage your stress. If you're interested in learning simple techniques to help you minimize stress, increase your energy and vitality, and increase your productivity, then write to me for more information on my new book"_

Master Keys to Health And Vtality , now available on Amazon in both Kindle and Paperback Formats.

(b) Although this might not be possible to work at a job you like at the moment, find aspects of the job that you're currently working at that you DO like. Write down at least 5 aspects or more, and keep them with you in your office or desk, so you can remind yourself of what you do like. Your "positive aspects list" is going to be an environmental cue, so whenever you see that list, you'll start to think of all things that you do like about that job. All you need to do is find just ONE, and then you'll start to notice others. Then, in the mean time, you can look around for employment that matches your interests and likes. Ask yourself:

"What's important to me in a job/career?" Have a pen and paper ready to record your answers. These are things that will help you to find that right job for YOU. Hey, the way I see it is this way: Life is too short to put yourself through something that you DON'T HAVE TO put yourself through. You don't have to walk around with 100 pound weights on each leg if you DON'T HAVE TO?

Would you kick yourself in the privates EVERYDAY if you DON'T HAVE TO? I certainly hope not. If your current Job is not offering you what it is you're looking to experience, then don't you owe it to yourself to find something does? While you're at that job that you don't really like too much, use your time WISELY and search for something that does. Is there a hobby that you're absolutely passionate about and you would actually pay to do it? If there was a way you could earn some money with that hobby, then what would that be...

But... when you do finally find something you truly love and something that fulfills you, then you can LOOK BACK and ask yourself:

"What did I learn about myself while I was working at xxx?"

What did I learn about others while I was working at xxx?"

It nice to have "a paycheck" coming in each week, but at the end of the day, is that really enough? Is all the pressure you're dealing worth the compensation? Again these are MY opinions and you either disagree or agree with me totally on this. Just remember:

You have the power to choose. Use your power. You purchased this manual because you CHOSE to see better.

C. Being happy with your family is crucial. If there are any issues/tension between you and members of your immediate family (people you live with or interact with on a daily basis), then sit down with them and talk things out, if possible. Even though words aren't exchanged, the tension is pretty damn loud. If possible, consider seeking professional help, such as a mediator to help you and the person(s) in question work things out. Emotions, both negative and positive, can build up inside of us like bubbles, and when they pop, hopefully they were filled with positive energy.

In most cases, being logical and rationally thinking through the situation will bring temporary relief. Really stop and think about the situation and the consequences of your desired actions. Focus on what you do want to happen in regards to said situation.

In conclusion, I'd just like to mention one thing, and it may seem like a no brainer for some of you, so please forgive me: The techniques in this manual will only work when you USE THEM. Just reading the manual and THINKING about the Tibetan eye chart included in this package will not improve your vision. Using and applying the knowledge therein will get your vision better and healthier.

Take Care and God Bless,

Amir K. Campbell

Make sure you sign up for my blog and get access to all the back posts with tons of useful information for your health, life, and success!!!

www.seathebiggerpicture.com

Follow me on instagram at amircampbell

Subscribe to my youtube channel for loads of FREE tips on health and fitness @ amircampbell

Bibliography

Bibliography/Recommended reading

1) Stone, Robert B. , *The Secret Life of Your Cells,* Pennsylvania: Whitford Press, 1989

2) Tracy, Brian, *Goals,* San Francisco, Berrett- Koehler publishers, Inc, 2003-2004

3) Esther and Jerry Hicks, *Money and the law of attraction*, United States: Hayhouse, 2008

4) Harold J. Reilly and Ruth hagy Brod, *The Edgar Cayce handbook for health through drugless therapy*, New York, McMillan Publishing Co: 1975

5) William S. Kroger and William D. Fezler, *Hypnosis and Behavior Modification: Imagery Conditioning*, Philadelphia, Toronto, J.B. Lippincott Co: 1976

6) Herbert Benson and Eileen M. Stuart, *The Wellness Book*, New York, Simon and Schuster, 1992

7) Donna Eden with David Feinstein, *Energy Medicine*, New York, Penguin Press Inc, 1998, 2008

8) Leslie M. LeCron, *Self Hypnotism: the technique and its use in Daily living*, New York, England, Penguin Group, 1970

9) Candace B. Pert, *Molecules of Emotion*, New York, Scribner, 2003

10) Linus Pauling, *How to Live Longer and Feel Better*, New York, Avon Books, 1986

11) Paul E. and Gail Dennison, *Brain gym Teacher's Edition*, California, Edu-kinesthetics, Inc, 1994

12) William H. Bates, *The Bates Method for Better Eyesight Without Glasses,* New York, Henry Holt and Company, 1940

Appendix A: A daily eye care plan you can follow in 5 minutes a day!!!

Daily Eye Rejuvenation Program

The Japanese are the perfect examples of "prevention, not cure". They developed a very effective eye care program for school children which calls for palming their eyes and then rubbing the orbits around the eye frequently throughout the day. This practice is surely a contributing factor in the lower rate of eye problems, including the need for glasses, found in Japanese children compared with children of the same age in the U.S.

Here's the program:

1) Upon waking, gently rub your eyes. This engages Stomach meridian and supports your eyes.

2) Palm your eyes while still in bed, and tap and rub the eye orbits to stimulate circulation.

3) Get yourself into the habit of attending to your eyes and their energies throughout the day. Give them new scenery and notice it. Shift from close vision to far vision, from focus to scanning. Keep your head moving and your eyes loose in your head.

4) Every so often, while you're reading or while working on the computer, rub around your eye sockets and then palm them for about a minute or so.

5) Do the "cover the eyes" (Palming) exercise several times during the day. This stimulates your peaceful circuits (your sympathetic nervous system) and helps to balance your triple

warmer and spleen meridians. It also helps bring flow and balance between the energies of your eyes and the rest of your body.

6) Figure 8 over your eyes. To make a figure 8, take your thumb, middle finger, and index finger and bunch them together. Pretend that you're weaving a pair of glasses over your eyes.

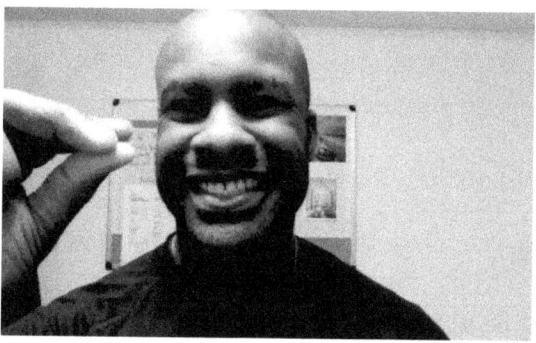

Fingers bunched together for weaving figure 8's over the eyes

7) Rinse glasses in cold water frequently.

8) Practice circling your eyes both counterclockwise and clockwise. Rotate them clockwise 15 times and then rotate them counterclockwise 15 times.

9) Practice drawing figure 8's in the air before you with your eyes. You'll notice that as you begin to practice, you may

have a challenging time making smooth figure 8's. However, with practice, your eyes will be able to make them easier and as a consequence, your vision will dramatically improve.

10) At various intervals during your day when you find time, simply close your eyes and remember something that makes you smile. This simple act will activate your relaxation response and give your eyes a rest when they need it.

11) Practice switching your focus back and forth between close objects and far out objects. This simple practice will help increase the flexibility of your eye lenses.

Appendix B

The Tibetan Eye Chart and How to use it to Improve Your Vision

I came across this little tool many years during my search for designing a preventive program for keeping my eyes strong and healthy. It's called the Tibetan Eye chart and it's purported to originate from Tibetan Buddhist temples. Whether or not this is the case, I don't know for sure, but I do know that using this simple tool in the way I'm going to describe will help you improve your vision in a very short time (when you combine it with all the other techniques in this book). It works by helping to increase the strength and flexibility of your lenses. It's very simple to use. To get the best results, make sure you remove your glasses or contacts.

Here's how:

1. Prepare your eyes by palming for about a minute.

2. Move your eyes clockwise around the circle, following the big circles at the edge.

3. Repeat the same motion going counterclockwise.

4. Focusing your vision on the center of the chart, move your eyes from the center up to the big circle at the 12 o clock position. Move your eyes back to center.

5. From the center position, move your eyes from there to the 2 o clock position. Once you get to the big dot, trace the line with your eyes back to the center.

6. Repeat this movement with all of the lines that have big circles on the end of them.

7. End this exercise by palming as in the beginning to rest them.

8. Go on about your day!!!

This regimen is best performed 2 times a day, once in the

morning before you start your day and once in the evening

before you get ready for bed.

Tibetan Eye Chart

Please print it out and place it on your wall for daily use.

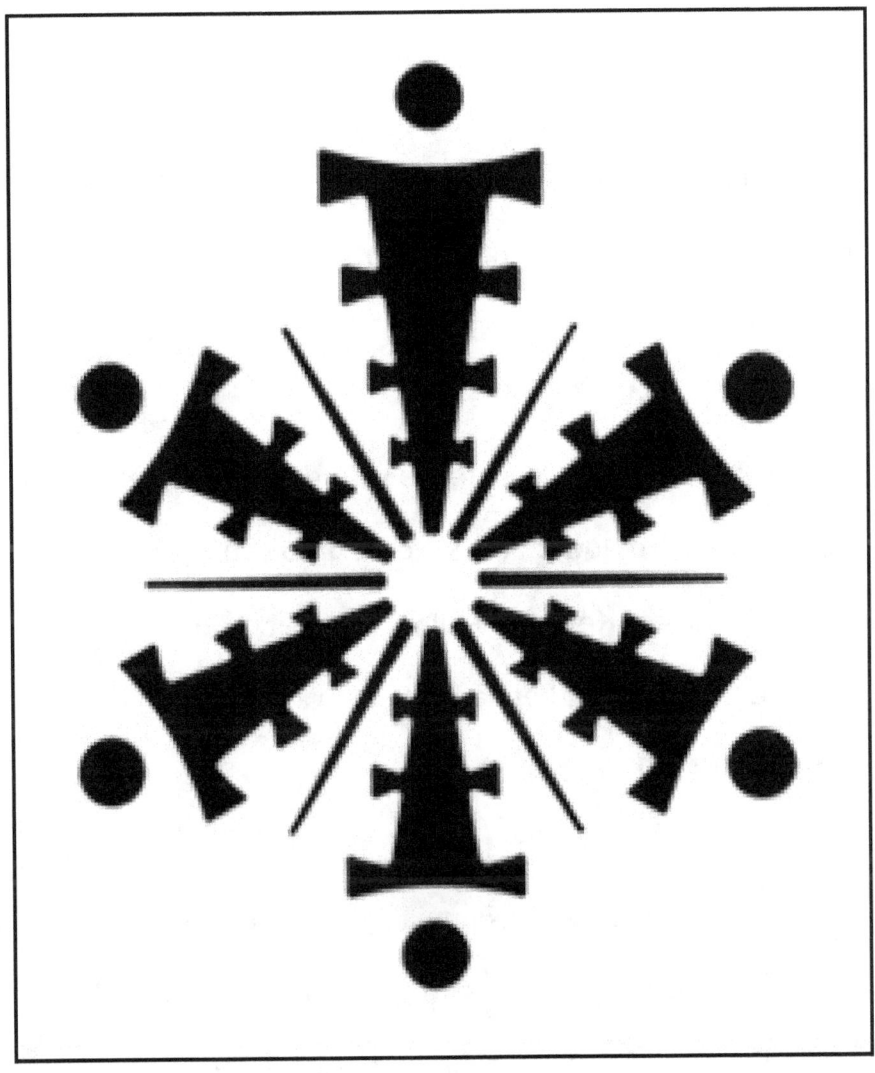

Afterword

Let me congratulate you again on taking a step to increase your personal power and improve your vision.

With consistent effort, you will experience better vision in 30 days or less.

If you want more ways to increase your energy and vitality and effectiveness and power in this world, grab your copy of my new book, Master Keys to Health and Vitality right now, available on Kindle and paperback. In this one-of-a-kind compendium, you'll learn:

o How to beat insomnia and sleep deeply!

o Age old tips to increase your sexual energy easily!

o Powerful mindfulness techniques to increase your perception of the world around!

o How to reduce anxiety and fear!

o A simple but POWERFUL technique to energize your organs and endocrine glands for maximum health!

o Powerful breathing techniques to send your vital force through the roof!

o Powerful ways to grow younger and vital by the day!!!

o How to eat to maximize youth promoting hormones!!

o How to design and LIVE the life you truly want!

o How to ease the symptoms of depression!

o Supplements to help increase your energy levels and burn excess fat like a furnace!

o How to run your mind for peak performance!

• How to know when to stop eating for maximum energy

• Relaxation techniques to relieve stress

• The signs of health and how you can change them

• The power of properly set intention

• The true value of exercise

• Why fresh air is better for you than you ever knew

• The value of proper eating

• How focusing on the positive is good for your health

- The influence of your thoughts on your body

- The Power of "I can..."

- The power in something so simple as a smile

- How imagination influences our bodies

- How our thoughts act as magnets

- What the ancient Taoists knew about the power of smiling

- Simple tips for better vision

- If you work in a office, then you'll thank me for this tip for quick and easy relaxation

- Bored at work? I'll share with you some tips for increasing your productivity and increasing your earning power

- A simple technique to relax you and energize you at the same time

- Need motivation to finish some project? Here's an incredibly simple drill to motivate yourself to accomplish virtually anything!

- Simple acupressure techniques to reduce stress INSTANTLY!!

- How to banish fear and program yourself to be brave instead!!!

o How to boost your immune system and mood in 30 seconds or less!!

You'll learn all of these and so much more!

Grab your copy today and experience unlimited health and vitality.

Go here now:

Master Keys To Health And Vitality

Master Keys to Health and Vitality

Amir K. Campbell

The Ultimate Guide To Optimal Health and Vitality

www.ingramcontent.com/pod-product-compliance
Lightning Source LLC
Chambersburg PA
CBHW062049280526
45788CB00003B/1156